Infused Water

Quick & Easy Vitamin Water Recipes for: Weight Loss, Detox & Fast Metabolism

2nd Edition–

Nick Bell

© **Copyright 2015 by Nick Bell. All rights reserved.**

This document is geared towards providing exact and reliable information in regards to the topic and issue covered. The publication is sold with the idea that the publisher is not required to render accounting, officially permitted, or otherwise, qualified services. If advice is necessary, legal or professional, a practiced individual in the profession should be ordered.

> - From the Declaration of Principles which was accepted and approved equally by the Committee of the American Bar Association and the Committee of Publishers and Associations.

In no way is it legal to reproduce, duplicate, or transmit any part of this document in either electronic means or in printed format. Recording of this publication is strictly prohibited and any storage of this document is not allowed unless with written permission from the publisher. All rights reserved.

The information provided herein is stated to be truthful and consistent, in that any liability, in terms of inattention or otherwise, by any usage or abuse of any policies, processes, or directions contained within is the solitary and utter responsibility of the recipient reader. Under no circumstances will any legal responsibility or blame be held against the publisher for any reparation, damages, or monetary loss due to the information herein, either directly or indirectly.

Respective authors own all copyrights not held by the publisher.

The information herein is offered for informational purposes solely, and is universal as so. The presentation of the information is without contract or any type of guarantee assurance.

The trademarks that are used are without any consent, and the publication of the trademark is without permission or backing by the trademark owner. All trademarks and brands within this book are for clarifying purposes only and are the owned by the owners themselves, not affiliated with this document.

Table of Contents

Introduction 1

Chapter 1. Water and Our Health 2

    Water Aids in Weight Loss 2

    Water Boosts Metabolism 3

    Water Detoxifies 3

    Harmful Drinks 3

    Fruit-Infused Vitamin Water 6

    Suggestions for Making Fruit-Infused Vitamin Water 7

Chapter 2: Benefits of Fruit Infused Water: 8

    Benefits of Fruit Infused Water: 8

Chapter 3. Mixed Fruit Recipes 11

    Blackberry Citrus 11

    Strawberry, Blueberry and Blackberry 12

    Cherry Lime 13

    Orange Pomegranate 14

    Raspberry Lime 15

    Strawberry Tangerine 16

    Apple Blueberry 16

    Strawberry Lime 17

    Triple Citrus 18

    Lemon Orange 19

    Blueberry Citrus 20

    Pineapple Orange 21

    Strawberry Lemon 22

    Blueberry Raspberry 23

    Pineapple, Apple and Grapefruit 23

Tropical Trio	24
Berry Cherry	25
Cantaloupe, Orange and Lemon	26
Berry Pomegranate	27
Raspberry Coconut	28
Kiwi Cucumber	29
Blueberry Peach Lemon	30
Coco-berry	31
Date Infused Water	31
Hibiscus, Star Fruit & Orange	32
Honeydew and Raspberry:	33
Berry Blast	33
Weight Watchers Drink	34
Grapefruit, Pineapple and Apple Water	35
Chapter 4. Spiced Water Recipes	**36**
Spiced Apple	36
Ginger Lemon	37
Strawberry Vanilla	38
Ginger Orange	39
Strawberry Jalapeno	39
Cucumber Lime with Basil and Mint	40
Watermelon Lime and Basil	41
Berry Spice	42
Rose Spice	43
Peach Vanilla	44
Cardamom, Vanilla and Orange	45
Watermelon-Jalapeno Cooler	46

Mango Ginger Delight	47
Raspberry, Rose Petal, and Vanilla	48
Spicy Orange Water	49
Fennel & Curry Leaves	50
Turmeric Ginger Tangerine	51
Spicy Concoction	52
Chapter 5. Herb Recipes	**54**
Basil, Cucumber and Lime	54
Rosemary and Friends	55
Mint and Cucumber	56
Blackberry and Sage	57
Rosemary and Watermelon	58
Mint, Basil, Lime and Cucumber	58
Rosemary, Orange and Lime	59
Orange Lavender	60
Mint, Plum, Apples and Blueberries	61
Sage Honeydew	62
Sage Berry	63
Nutmeg Cranapple	64
Lavender Kiwi	65
Cinnamon Apple	66
Pineapple Thyme	67
Cranberry, Orange and Mint	67
Grapefruit, Sage and Strawberries	68
Rosy Cukes	69
Blueberry, Orange and Basil	70
Basil Mango	71

Strawberry Cucumber Basil	72
Lemongrass Mint	73
Pineapple-Strawberry Cooler	73
Rosemary and Grapefruit	74
True Blue	74
Vanilla Basil Strawberry	75
Fennel & Pear	76
Blueberry Cucumber & Basil	76
Orange Lavender	77
Raspberry & Rose	78
Mango Pineapple Mint	79
Chapter 6. Minced Herb Recipes	**80**
Citrus, Basil and Mint	80
Mint, Cucumber and Lemon	81
Berry and Sage	82
Mint Pineapple	83
Basil, Kiwi and Strawberry	83
Rosemary, Grapefruit and Orange	84
Mint, Lime and Watermelon	85
Tarragon, Lime and Cherry	86
Thyme, Peach and Blueberry	87
Mint Peach	88
Tropical Mince herbed water	89
Green apple Raspberry Rosemary	90
Kiwi Blackberry Thyme & Basil	91
Root Delight	92
Black Lady	92

Carrot Cooler	93
Chapter 7. More Recipes	**94**
Cucumber Citrus	94
Pineapple Cucumber	95
Strawberry Chamomile	96
Cucumber Lemon	96
Ginger Tea	97
Cucumber Melon	98
Strawberry, Cucumber and Citrus	99
Blood Orange	100
Hibiscus Watermelon	101
Conclusion	**102**
Recipe Sources Used in this Book	**103**
Breakfast Recipes	**106**
Cinnamon French Toast	106
Check Out My Other Books	**109**
Offer for Free Books	**110**
One Last Thing	**111**

Introduction

I want to thank you and congratulate you for downloading the book, *Fruit-Infused Vitamin Water: Over 70 Quick and Easy Vitamin Water Recipes for Weight Loss, Detox and Metabolism Boosting.*

How many glasses of water do you drink every day? It is no secret that water is essential for to our survival. Water is abundant, yet we sometimes take it for granted. Our body is two-thirds water, and we would not last without it for a few days.

Do you know that drinking at least eight glasses of water daily can decrease the risk of bladder cancer by 50%, colon cancer by 45% and even potentially reduce the risk of other ailments? This is because it helps in ridding our bodies of toxins we get from the environment and the food we eat. Hydrating does so many benefits for us that it makes sense to include natural vitamins in our drinking water to maximize its health potential.

This book contains quick recipes for delicious fruit-infused vitamin water that has demonstrated its potential to help people lose weight, boost their metabolic rates and rid their bodies of dangerous toxins. Our recipes also provide you with an energy boost and loads of vitamins, minerals and other essential nutrients. The best thing about our recipes is that it is all-natural and homemade. It means it gives you 100% of the health benefits without adding any calories, refined sugar or chemical additives.

Thanks again for downloading this book, I hope you enjoy it!

Chapter 1.
Water and Our Health

Just how important is water for our health? Water makes up 2/3 of our body weight and is distributed in vital organs of the body; the human brain is 95% water, the lungs 90%, and our blood 82%. Just a 2% drop in our body's water supply can trigger signs of dehydration like fatigue, lack of focus, and fuzzy short-term memory.

Just as a car cannot run without gas and oil, the body cannot work without water. All organ functions depend on water for their proper functioning – from digestion, perspiration, movement (lubricating the joints), to regulating the body temperature. Most importantly, water is the medium in eliminating waste and toxins from our bodies.

Water Aids in Weight Loss

A study conducted by researchers at Virginia Tech found that dieters who increased their water intake between meals for a period of twelve weeks lost about five pounds more than those who didn't. One theory behind this is that the increased water consumption makes dieters feel fuller and consequently eat less. And of course, drinking more water leads to drinking less of other fluids, most of which contain calories.

Water Boosts Metabolism

Drinking water also speeds up metabolism (your body's ability to burn fat). Scientific tests found that drinking about 17oz of water increases metabolic rate by 30% in healthy men and women. This boost happened within 10 minutes of drinking water, but reached a maximum 30-40 minutes after drinking.

Water Detoxifies

Water absorbs (and eliminates) more toxins from your body than commercial fruit juices do, because water is pure, containing nothing else. Fruit juices are largely saturated with fruit, sugars, and other substances, so they simply aren't able to absorb much more substance, much as a wet sponge can't absorb any more dirt.

Fruit-infused vitamin water, on the other hand, offers the best of both worlds, offering much of the same nutrients that fruit juices provide, while being pure enough to absorb a lot of toxins.

Harmful Drinks

Most drinks you buy these days contain additives that are harmful to our health. When I found out about the health hazards of commercial beverages, I decided to stop buying these and started making fruit-infused water for my family, and we haven't turned back. In fact, we can't get enough of the stuff. It's the healthier and cheaper alternative!

Here are a few of the facts about commercial beverages, facts that make me cringe every time I think of what my family and I used to drink.

Diet Soda Pop

A study of almost ten thousand people conducted by the University of Minnesota found that one diet soda a day was linked to a 34% higher risk of metabolic syndrome. Symptoms include belly fat and high cholesterol that put people at risk for heart disease.

A research study by the University of Texas found that drinking two or more cans a day of diet pop increased weight gain by 500%. Why? The reason for it might be that artificial sweeteners can disrupt our body's ability to regulate caloric intake. The artificial sweeteners trick us into thinking we're eating sugar, which makes us crave more sugar, leading to overeating, as a study by Purdue University suggested.

Unlike regular soda pops, most diet pops contain mold inhibitors like sodium benzoate and potassium benzoate. "These chemicals have the ability to cause severe damage to DNA in the mitochondria to the point that they totally inactivate it—they knock it out altogether," says Peter Piper, a professor of molecular biology at the University of Sheffield in the UK. The Center for Science in the Public Interest says these preservatives also have been linked to allergies like asthma and hives.

A study by the Harvard Medical School of more than three thousand women associated drinking more than two diet pops a day had a two-fold risk of declining kidney function.

Regular Soda Pop
All regular and diet soda pop cans are coated with bisophenol-A (BPA), which researchers have linked to numerous ailments, including reproductive problems, obesity, and heart disease. Regular soda pop is also high in phosphoric acid, which can contribute to osteoporosis and weak bones.

The high acidity of both regular and diet pop dissolves tooth enamel, leading to cavities. In regular pop, this acidity combined with caffeine has been shown to raise the acidic level of the stomach, leading to gastrointestinal problems. Additionally, soda pop can contribute to caffeine addiction and its associated problems.

One can of soda pop contains approximately the recommended daily limit of sugar intake, so any other sugar consumed in the day might as well contribute to obesity, diabetes and a host of other health risks.

Energy Drinks and Coffee
The caffeine in energy drinks; coffee and soda pop can elevate blood pressure, which can lead to an increased risk of stroke, cerebral vascular disease, insomnia, hallucinations, Parkinson's disease, diabetes, cardiovascular diseases and dementia.

According to Robert Tozzi, chief of pediatric cardiology at Hackensack University Medical Center in New Jersey, "Energy drinks are not safe, and do not improve performance. Water is your best fluid."

Sports Drinks
Most sports drinks are loaded with harmful stuff like sodium, calories, refined sugar and artificial ingredients. The selling

point for these sports drinks is that they contain electrolytes. But according to Fit Day.com, these electrolytes are rarely necessary. "Even after completing such endurance sports as a marathon or a triathlon, most individuals can properly recover their body's electrolytes with food rather than drink. By eating a healthy, balanced meal after a strenuous workout, you can ensure you're not consuming excess sugar through sports drinks. Instead, properly hydrate with a cool glass of water."

If there's one thing that nutritionists agree upon, it's that refined sugar is bad for you. The issues with sugar include the increased risks of diabetes, cancer, pancreatic burnout, liver problems, obesity, high blood pressure, accelerated aging, sugar addiction, cognitive decline and a host of other ailments.

Fruit-Infused Vitamin Water

Proper hydration through drinking homemade fruit-infused water helps to maintain your proper heart rate, body temperature and blood pressure, and also helps rid your body of excess salts. Homemade fruit-infused water does all this without any calories, refined sugar or chemical additives.

Our quick recipes for delicious fruit-infused vitamin water have been demonstrated to help people lose weight, boost their metabolic rates and rid their bodies of dangerous toxins. Our recipes also provide you with an energy boost and loads of vitamins, minerals and other essential nutrients.

Suggestions for Making Fruit-Infused Vitamin Water

Use your favorite drinking water, whether it's filtered, ionized, reverse osmosis, spring or distilled. You can also use sparkling water, though it goes flat quickly, or unsweetened carbonated water.

Glass mason jars and pitchers are nice because plastic absorbs and holds flavors, even after repeated washings. You might want to use plastic lids for the mason jars, though, to avoid the potential rust from metal lids. Sprout topper lids work well for straining mason jars. You can also buy fruit-infused water pitchers, which are handy.

Wooden muddlers are nice for pressing the fruit, though wooden spoons work okay. Muddlers are available from various online shops like Amazon.

The longer you let your infused water sit before using it, the stronger the flavor will be. But remember that the water should be refrigerated and consumed within a maximum of two or three days to ensure freshness and maximize the benefits.

Many people like to use the same batch of fruit two or three times, so they only let it soak for a few hours for each batch and then drink the batch within one day. Some people make strong batches and then let people dilute it to their individual tastes.

Chapter 2:
Benefits of Fruit Infused Water:

Benefits of Fruit Infused Water:

A lot of people do not enjoy drinking water, for a simple reason that it tastes too plain to excite your taste buds. Well, it may not have any taste but has ample benefits. If you drink less water, you can get dehydrated, which in turn gives rise to different types of illness. Dehydration in the long run can cause joint pains, dizziness, obesity, headaches etc. To avoid all these issues, you have to drink water. So, to make it more interesting and give your pain old glass of water a cool twist, we bring to you fruit infused water.

There are numerous health benefits of drinking fruit infused water; some of them are as below

- Purifies the body and flushes out the toxins
- You get more vitamin contents than fresh fruit juice
- Filled with natural antioxidants, vitamins and minerals
- Much less sugar content and in turn calories, as compared to natural fruit juice.
- Increases concentration
- Increases metabolism
- Increases productivity

- Gives you a glowing skin thereby improving your complexion. Keeps your skin elastic and supple.

- Helps in weight loss

- Proper functioning of kidneys by sending wastes through urine

- It flushes your entire system. Waste is sent out of the body through sweating and bowel movements.

- Maintains high energy levels in your body throughout the day. You will not feel tired and sleepy, which general weight loss diets will make you feel.

- Helps you keep yourself hydrated while exercising. Lowers the muscle tiredness. It helps you to recover faster after your work out. Better than having energy drinks which give you unnecessary empty calories

- Helps you with your mood swings (from bad to good)

- Maintains healthy organs

- Maintains good bone health by lubricating joints

- Delays appearance of wrinkles

A few know how's of fruit infused water:

- Infuse the water for about 2-3 hours for a milder flavor and color. Infusing for longer time gives better flavor and color to the water. Best infused at room temperature for 3 hours and then refrigerated for a few more hours. Do not consume infused water that is placed at room temperature for more than 4-5 hours as bacteria can set in.

- To store the infused water in the refrigerator after infusing, make sure you remove the fruits and herbs or whatever ingredients you have added to infuse. Otherwise the ingredients may rot.

- Do not store the infused water for long. Store for not more than 3 days. The fresher the infused water, the better.

- It is best not to add the rinds of lemon, limes, orange, tangerine, and mandarin etc. as it tends to be bitter. If you have to, then do not infuse for more than 3 hours or best just squeeze these fruits in the water.

- It is best to consume your infused water at room temperate or cold, try not to drink hot water.

- Fresh fruits infuse better than frozen fruits. Dry fruits do not give a good taste so it is better not to use dry fruits.

- It best to use glass jars for infusing. Infused water pitchers are also available for making larger quantities. For lesser quantities, masons jars are perfect.

Chapter 3.
Mixed Fruit Recipes

These recipes call for various combinations of straight fruit, without any herbs or spices. These delicious and tested recipes are perfect for hot summer days when fruit is simply the most abundant natural food in the world to eat.

Blackberry Citrus

Ingredients:

- 2 slices orange
- 3 slices lime
- 10 blackberries

Directions:

1. Put all the fruits into a one-quart glass jar and press with a wooden spoon or muddler, twisting it slightly until the fruit begins to release its juices. Don't pulverize the fruit into pieces.

2. If you plan to drink all or most of the fruit water within the next five hours, fill the jar halfway with ice and then top the jar off with cold drinking water. If you're planning to store the water for longer than five hours before drinking it, fill the jar three-quarters full of ice before topping it off with water.

3. Stir with a chopstick or long spoon and put a lid on the jar. Stick the jar in the fridge to chill, preferably for at least three hours.

4. Strain the water before serving.

Strawberry, Blueberry and Blackberry

This combo offers a light and delicious berry flavor that is packed with antioxidants.

Ingredients:

- 4 strawberries
- 10 blueberries
- 10 blackberries

Directions:

1. Put all the fruits into a one-quart glass jar and press with a wooden spoon or muddler, twisting it slightly until the fruit begins to release its juices. Don't pulverize the fruit into pieces.

2. If you plan to drink all or most of the fruit water within the next five hours, fill the jar halfway with ice and then top the jar off with cold drinking water. If you're planning to store the water for longer than five hours before drinking it, fill the jar three-quarters full of ice before topping it off with water.

3. Stir with a chopstick or long spoon and put a lid on the jar. Stick the jar in the fridge to chill, preferably for at least three hours.

4. Strain the water before serving.

Cherry Lime

Ingredients:

- 12 cherries
- ½ lime, peeled and sliced

Directions:

1. Remove the pits from the cherries. Put the cherries and lime into a one-quart glass jar and press them with a wooden spoon or muddler, twisting it slightly until the fruit begins to release its juices. Don't pulverize the fruit into pieces.

2. If you plan to drink all or most of the fruit water within the next five hours, fill the jar halfway with ice and then top the jar off with cold drinking water. If you're planning to store the water for longer than five hours before drinking it, fill the jar three-quarters full of ice before topping it off with water.

3. Stir with a chopstick or long spoon and put a lid on the jar. Stick the jar in the fridge to chill, preferably for at least three hours.

4. Strain the water before serving.

Orange Pomegranate

Ingredients:

- 2 oranges, peeled and sliced
- ½ cup pomegranate seeds

Directions:

1. Put the oranges and pomegranate seeds into a one-quart glass jar and press the fruits with a wooden spoon or muddler, twisting it slightly until the fruit begins to release its juices. Don't pulverize the fruit into pieces.

2. If you plan to drink all or most of the fruit water within the next five hours, fill the jar halfway with ice and then top the jar off with cold drinking water. If you're planning to store the water for longer than five hours before drinking it, fill the jar three-quarters full of ice before topping it off with water.

3. Stir with a chopstick or long spoon and put a lid on the jar. Stick the jar in the fridge to chill, preferably for at least three hours.

4. Strain the water before serving.

Raspberry Lime

Ingredients:

- 2 limes

- 20 raspberries

Directions:

1. Quarter the limes and squeeze the juice with your hands into a two-quart glass jar or pitcher and then toss the squeezed quarters in with the juice.

2. Add the raspberries and press them with a wooden spoon or muddler, twisting it slightly until the raspberries begin to release their juice. Don't pulverize the fruit into pieces.

3. If you plan to drink all or most of the fruit water within the next five hours, fill the jar halfway with ice and then top the jar off with cold drinking water. If you're planning to store the water for longer than five hours before drinking it, fill the jar three-quarters full of ice before topping it off with water.

4. Stir with a chopstick or long spoon and put a lid on the jar. Stick the jar in the fridge to chill, preferably for at least three hours.

5. Strain the water before serving.

Strawberry Tangerine

Ingredients:

- ¾ cup sliced strawberries
- 1 tangerine rind

Directions:

- Remove the white pith from the rind. Put the rind and strawberries into a one-quart glass jar and press the fruits with a wooden spoon or muddler, twisting it slightly until the fruit begins to release its juices. Don't pulverize the fruit into pieces.

- If you plan to drink all or most of the fruit water within the next five hours, fill the jar halfway with ice and then top the jar off with cold drinking water. If you're planning to store the water for longer than five hours before drinking it, fill the jar three-quarters full of ice before topping it off with water.

- Stir with a chopstick or long spoon and put a lid on the jar. Stick the jar in the fridge to chill, preferably for at least three hours.

- Strain the water before serving.

Apple Blueberry

Ingredients:

- ½ cup blueberries

- 1 apple, cored and sliced thinly

Directions:

1. Put the blueberries into a one-quart glass jar and press them with a wooden spoon or muddler, twisting it slightly until the fruit begins to release its juices. Don't pulverize the fruit into pieces. Add the apples without muddling them.

2. If you plan to drink all or most of the fruit water within the next five hours, fill the jar halfway with ice and then top the jar off with cold drinking water. If you're planning to store the water for longer than five hours before drinking it, fill the jar three-quarters full of ice before topping it off with water.

3. Stir with a chopstick or long spoon and put a lid on the jar. Stick the jar in the fridge to chill, preferably for at least three hours.

4. Strain the water before serving.

Strawberry Lime

Ingredients:

- 8 strawberries
- 3 slices of lime

Directions:

1. Quarter the limes and squeeze the juice with your hands into a two-quart glass jar or pitcher and then toss the squeezed quarters in with the juice.

2. Add the strawberries and press them with a wooden spoon or muddler, twisting it slightly until the strawberries begin to release their juice. Don't pulverize the fruit into pieces.

3. If you plan to drink all or most of the fruit water within the next five hours, fill the jar halfway with ice and then top the jar off with cold drinking water. If you're planning to store the water for longer than five hours before drinking it, fill the jar three-quarters full of ice before topping it off with water.

4. Stir with a chopstick or long spoon and put a lid on the jar. Stick the jar in the fridge to chill, preferably for at least three hours.

5. Strain the water before serving.

Triple Citrus

Ingredients:

- 1 orange
- 1 lime
- 1 lemon

Directions:

1. Slice the orange, lime and lemon each into rounds and then cut the rounds in half. Put the pieces of fruit into a two-quart glass jar or pitcher. Press the slices with a wooden spoon or muddler, twisting it slightly until the fruit begins releasing its juices. Don't press so much that you pulverize the fruit into pieces.

2. If you plan to drink all or most of the fruit water within the next five hours, fill the jar halfway with ice and then top the jar off with cold drinking water. If you're planning to store the water for longer than five hours before drinking it, fill the jar three-quarters full of ice and then top the jar off with water.

3. Stir with a chopstick or long spoon and put a lid on the jar. Stick the jar in the fridge to chill, preferably for at least three hours.

4. Strain the water before serving.

Lemon Orange

Ingredients:

- 3 mandarin oranges
- 1 lemon, sliced

Directions:

1. Put the oranges and lemon into a one-quart glass jar and press them with a wooden spoon or muddler,

twisting it slightly until the fruit begins to release its juices. Don't pulverize the fruit into pieces.

2. If you plan to drink all or most of the fruit water within the next five hours, fill the jar halfway with ice and then top the jar off with cold drinking water. If you're planning to store the water for longer than five hours before drinking it, fill the jar three-quarters full of ice before topping it off with water.

3. Stir with a chopstick or long spoon and put a lid on the jar. Stick the jar in the fridge to chill, preferably for at least three hours.

4. Strain the water before serving.

Blueberry Citrus

Ingredients:

- 10 blueberries
- 1 lemon slice
- 2 orange slices

Directions:

1. Put all the fruits into a one-quart glass jar and press with a wooden spoon or muddler, twisting it slightly until the fruit begins to release its juices. Don't pulverize the fruit into pieces.

2. If you plan to drink all or most of the fruit water within the next five hours, fill the jar halfway with ice and then top the jar off with cold drinking water. If you're planning to store the water for longer than five hours before drinking it, fill the jar three-quarters full of ice before topping it off with water.

3. Stir with a chopstick or long spoon and put a lid on the jar. Stick the jar in the fridge to chill, preferably for at least three hours.

4. Strain the water before serving.

Pineapple Orange

Ingredients:

- 1 orange, peeled and sliced
- ½ c. pineapple, cut into bite-sized chunks

Directions:

1. Put the orange slices and pineapple chunks into a one-quart glass jar and press them with a wooden spoon or muddler, twisting it slightly until the fruit begins to release its juices. Don't pulverize the fruit into pieces.

2. If you plan to drink all or most of the fruit water within the next five hours, fill the jar halfway with ice and then top the jar off with cold drinking water. If you're planning to store the water for longer than five hours before drinking it, fill the jar three-quarters full of ice before topping it off with water.

3. Stir with a chopstick or long spoon and put a lid on the jar. Stick the jar in the fridge to chill, preferably for at least three hours.

4. Strain the water before serving.

Strawberry Lemon

Ingredients:

- 15 strawberries, topped and sliced
- 1 lemon, peeled and sliced

Directions:

1. Put all the fruits into a one-quart glass jar and press them with a wooden spoon or muddler, twisting it slightly until the fruit begins to release its juices. Don't pulverize the fruit into pieces.

2. If you plan to drink all or most of the fruit water within the next five hours, fill the jar halfway with ice and then top the jar off with cold drinking water. If you're planning to store the water for longer than five hours before drinking it, fill the jar three-quarters full of ice before topping it off with water.

3. Stir with a chopstick or long spoon and put a lid on the jar. Stick the jar in the fridge to chill, preferably for at least three hours.

4. Strain the water before serving.

Blueberry Raspberry

Ingredients:

- ½ cup blueberries
- 5 raspberries

Directions:

1. Put all the berries into a one-quart glass jar and press them with a wooden spoon or muddler, twisting it slightly until the fruit begins to release its juices. Don't pulverize the fruit into pieces.

2. If you plan to drink all or most of the fruit water within the next five hours, fill the jar halfway with ice and then top the jar off with cold drinking water. If you're planning to store the water for longer than five hours before drinking it, fill the jar three-quarters full of ice before topping it off with water.

3. Stir with a chopstick or long spoon and put a lid on the jar. Stick the jar in the fridge to chill, preferably for at least three hours.

4. Strain the water before serving.

Pineapple, Apple and Grapefruit

Ingredients:

- ½ apple, sliced

- 1 cup pineapple chunks

- ½ grapefruit, peeled and sliced

Directions:

1. Put all the fruits into a one-quart glass jar and press them with a wooden spoon or muddler, twisting it slightly until the fruit begins to release its juices. Don't pulverize the fruit into pieces.

2. If you plan to drink all or most of the fruit water within the next five hours, fill the jar halfway with ice and then top the jar off with cold drinking water. If you're planning to store the water for longer than five hours before drinking it, fill the jar three-quarters full of ice before topping it off with water.

3. Stir with a chopstick or long spoon and put a lid on the jar. Stick the jar in the fridge to chill, preferably for at least three hours.

4. Strain the water before serving.

Tropical Trio

Ingredients:

- ½ quart coconut water

- 1 cup pineapple chunks

- ½ cup mango chunks

Directions:

1. Put all the pineapple and mango chunks into a one-quart glass jar and press it with a wooden spoon or muddler, twisting it slightly until the fruit begins to release its juices. Don't pulverize the fruit into pieces.

2. Fill the glass jar with the coconut water. If you plan to drink all or most of the fruit water within the next five hours, fill the jar halfway with ice and then top the jar off with cold drinking water.

3. Stir with a chopstick or long spoon and put a lid on the jar. Stick the jar in the fridge to chill, preferably for at least three hours.

4. Strain the water before serving.

Berry Cherry

Ingredients:

- ½ cup blueberries
- ½ cup raspberries
- ½ cup cherries

Directions:

1. Put all the fruits into a one-quart glass jar and press them with a wooden spoon or muddler, twisting it slightly until the fruit begins to release its juices. Don't pulverize the fruit into pieces.

2. If you plan to drink all or most of the fruit water within the next five hours, fill the jar halfway with ice and then top the jar off with cold drinking water. If you're planning to store the water for longer than five hours before drinking it, fill the jar three-quarters full of ice before topping it off with water.

3. Stir with a chopstick or long spoon and put a lid on the jar. Stick the jar in the fridge to chill, preferably for at least three hours.

4. Strain the water before serving.

Cantaloupe, Orange and Lemon

Ingredients:

- ½ cantaloupe, cut into chunks
- 1 blood orange, peeled and sliced
- 1 lemon, peeled and sliced

Directions:

1. Put the fruits into a one-quart glass jar and press it with a wooden spoon or muddler, twisting it slightly until the fruit begins to release its juices. Don't pulverize the fruit into pieces.

2. If you plan to drink all or most of the fruit water within the next five hours, fill the jar halfway with ice and then top the jar off with cold drinking water. If you're planning to store the water for longer than five hours

before drinking it, fill the jar three-quarters full of ice before topping it off with water.

3. Stir with a chopstick or long spoon and put a lid on the jar. Stick the jar in the fridge to chill, preferably for at least three hours.

4. Strain the water before serving.

Berry Pomegranate

You can use all the seeds from a pomegranate for this.

Ingredients:

- 1 pomegranate worth of seeds
- ½ cup blueberries
- ½ cup raspberries

Directions:

1. Put all the berries into a one-quart glass jar and press them with a wooden spoon or muddler, twisting the muddler slightly until the fruit begins to release its juices. Don't pulverize the fruit into pieces. Add the pomegranate seeds.

2. If you plan to drink all or most of the fruit water within the next five hours, fill the jar halfway with ice and then top the jar off with cold drinking water. If you're planning to store the water for longer than five hours

before drinking it, fill the jar three-quarters full of ice before topping it off with water.

3. Stir with a chopstick or long spoon and put a lid on the jar. Stick the jar in the fridge to chill, preferably for at least three hours.

4. Strain the water before serving.

Raspberry Coconut

Ingredients:

- ½ quart coconut water
- ½ c. raspberries
- 2 slices lemon

Directions:

1. Put the raspberries into a one-quart glass jar and press it with a wooden spoon or muddler, twisting it slightly until the fruit begins to release its juices. Don't pulverize the fruit into pieces. Squeeze the lemon, adding the juice and the lemon slice to the mixture. Finally, add the ½ quart coconut water.

2. If you plan to drink all or most of the fruit water within the next five hours, fill the jar halfway with ice and then top the jar off with cold drinking water.

3. Stir with a chopstick or long spoon and put a lid on the jar. Stick the jar in the fridge to chill, preferably for at least three hours.

4. Strain the water before serving.

Kiwi Cucumber

Ingredients:

- 3 kiwis, peeled, sliced thinly
- 1 small cucumber, peeled, seeded, sliced

Directions:

1. Put the kiwis and cucumber slices into a one-quart glass jar and press with a wooden spoon or muddle, twisting it slightly until the fruit begins to release its juices. Don't pulverize the fruit into pieces.

2. If you plan to drink all or most of the fruit water within the next five hours, fill the jar halfway with ice and then top the jar off with cold drinking water. If you're planning to store the water for longer than five hours before drinking it, fill the jar three-quarters full of ice before topping it off with water.

3. Stir with a chopstick or long spoon and put a lid on the jar. Stick the jar in the fridge to chill, preferably for at least three hours.

4. Strain the water before serving.

Blueberry Peach Lemon

Ingredients:

- ½ cup blueberries
- 3 slices lemon
- 5-6 peach slices
- 8-10 mint leaves

Directions:

1. Put all the fruits into a one-quart glass jar and press with a wooden spoon or muddle, twisting it slightly until the fruit begins to release its juices. Don't pulverize the fruit into pieces.

2. If you plan to drink all or most of the fruit water within the next five hours, fill the jar halfway with ice and then top the jar off with cold drinking water. If you're planning to store the water for longer than five hours before drinking it, fill the jar three-quarters full of ice before topping it off with water.

3. Stir with a chopstick or long spoon and put a lid on the jar. Stick the jar in the fridge to chill, preferably for at least three hours.

4. Strain the water before serving.

Coco-berry

Ingredients:

- ½ cup blueberries
- ½ cup blackberries
- 1 peach, pitted, cut into half-inch wedges
- 3 cups spring or filtered water
- 1 cup coconut water
- 1 clean glass jar with lid

Directions:

1. Add the berries to the jar. Place the peach over the berries. Pour water and coconut water. Stir with a chopstick or a long spoon.
2. Refrigerate for a minimum of 3-4 hours.
3. Strain the water before serving.

Date Infused Water

Ingredients:

- 3 cups raspberries
- 12 cups spring or filtered water
- 2 large lemons, cut into half-inch slices

- 4 dried Medjool dates, pitted, chopped
- 1 large clean glass jar with lid

Directions:

1. Add raspberries to the bottom of the jar. Layer with dates followed by lemon slices.
2. Pour water and stir well. Fasten the lid.
3. Refrigerate for an hour. Strain and serve the infused water.

Hibiscus, Star Fruit & Orange

Ingredients:

- 7-8 hibiscus flowers (petals only)
- 6 slices orange
- 6 slices star fruit
- 10 glasses water

Direction:

1. Boil about 4 glasses of water. Remove from heat. Add the hibiscus petals. Cover and keep aside to cool.
2. Meanwhile add to a large glass jar the rest of the ingredients. Close the lid. Refrigerate for 2-3 hours.

3. When the hibiscus tea cools down, strain and discard the petals. Add to the glass jar. Stir well' Let it infuse for at least an hour.

4. Strain and serve the infused water.

Honeydew and Raspberry:

Ingredients:

- 5-6 slices honeydew
- 1 lime, sliced
- 1 cup raspberries
- 6 glasses water

Directions:

1. Add all the ingredients to a glass jar. Stir well. Fasten the lid.
2. Refrigerate for 2-3 hours. Strain and serve the infused water.

Berry Blast

Ingredients:

- ½ cup blueberries
- ½ cup blackberries

- ½ cup strawberries, sliced
- ½ cup raspberries
- ½ cup pomegranate seeds
- 8 cups water

Directions:

1. Add all the ingredients to a glass jar. Stir well. Fasten the lid.
2. Refrigerate for 2-3 hours. Strain and serve the infused water.

Weight Watchers Drink

Ingredients:

- 4 cups green tea, brewed
- 5-6 slices tangerine
- 8-10 mint leaves

Directions:

1. Add all the ingredients to a glass jar. Stir well. Fasten the lid.
2. Refrigerate for 4-5 hours. Strain and serve the infused water.

Grapefruit, Pineapple and Apple Water

Ingredients:

- 1 grapefruit, peeled, seeded, sliced
- 1 apple, cored, sliced
- 1 fresh pineapple, peeled, cored, sliced
- Water as required

Directions:

1. Add all the ingredients to a large glass jar. Stir well. Fasten the lid.
2. Refrigerate for 4-5 hours. Strain and serve the infused water.
3. When half of your jar is empty, fill with some more water. This can be repeated a couple of times.

Chapter 4.
Spiced Water Recipes

These recipes include one or more spices, along with fruit. They're perfect for evenings when you're snuggling around the fireplace, wanting a little extra spice in your life.

Spiced Apple

Ingredients:

- 1 apple, sliced
- 1 cinnamon stick or 1 piece of cinnamon bark
- 6 whole cloves
- 3 whole pieces of nutmeg

Directions:

1. Put all the ingredients into a two-quart glass jar or pitcher. If you plan to drink all or most of the fruit water within the next eight hours, fill the jar halfway with ice and then top the jar off with cold drinking water.

2. If you're planning to store the water for longer than eight hours before drinking it, fill the jar three-quarters full of ice before topping it off with water.

3. Stick the jar in the fridge to chill, preferably for at least six hours.

4. Strain the water before serving.

Ginger Lemon

Ingredients:

- ½ lemon, sliced

- 3-inch chunk of ginger, peeled and cut up

Directions:

1. Put the lemon into a one-quart glass jar and press it lightly with a muddle or a wooden spoon, twisting the muddle enough to start releasing the fruit juices. Don't pulverize the lemon into pieces. Add the cut-up ginger.

2. If you plan to drink all or most of the fruit water within the next five hours, fill the jar halfway with ice and then top the jar off with cold drinking water. If you're planning to store the water for longer than five hours before drinking it, fill the jar three-quarters full of ice before topping it off with water.

3. Stir with a chopstick or long spoon and put a lid on the jar. Stick the jar in the fridge to chill, preferably for at least three hours.

4. Strain the water before serving.

Strawberry Vanilla

Ingredients:

- 10 strawberries, tops removed and sliced
- 1 vanilla bean, sliced lengthwise

Directions:

1. Put the strawberries into a one-quart glass jar and press them with a muddle or a wooden spoon, twisting the muddle to start releasing the fruit juices. Don't pulverize the strawberries into pieces.

2. Scrape the vanilla out of the bean and add it to the jar. You can optionally also add the bean itself to the jar.

3. If you plan to drink all or most of the fruit water within the next five hours, fill the jar halfway with ice and then top the jar off with cold drinking water. If you're planning to store the water for longer than five hours before drinking it, fill the jar three-quarters full of ice before topping it off with water.

4. Stir with a chopstick or long spoon and put a lid on the jar. Stick the jar in the fridge to chill, preferably for at least three hours.

5. Strain the water before serving.

Ginger Orange

Ingredients:

- 1 small piece of ginger
- 1 orange, peeled and sliced

Directions:

1. Skin the ginger and slice it into small rings. Put it into a one-quart glass jar and press it lightly with a muddle or a wooden spoon. Add the orange slices and press them, twisting them enough to start releasing the fruit juices. Don't pulverize the herbs or fruit into pieces.

2. If you plan to drink all or most of the fruit water within the next five hours, fill the jar halfway with ice and then top the jar off with cold drinking water. If you're planning to store the water for longer than five hours before drinking it, fill the jar three-quarters full of ice before topping it off with water.

3. Stir with a chopstick or long spoon and put a lid on the jar. Stick the jar in the fridge to chill, preferably for at least three hours.

4. Strain the water before serving.

Strawberry Jalapeno

Ingredients:

- 10 strawberries, with tops removed

- ¼ of a jalapeno pepper

Directions:

1. Put the strawberries and jalapeno into a one-quart glass jar and press them lightly with a muddle or a wooden spoon, twisting the muddle enough to start releasing the fruit juices. Don't pulverize the fruit into pieces.

2. If you plan to drink all or most of the fruit water within the next five hours, fill the jar halfway with ice and then top the jar off with cold drinking water. If you're planning to store the water for longer than five hours before drinking it, fill the jar three-quarters full of ice before topping it off with water.

3. Stir with a chopstick or long spoon and put a lid on the jar. Stick the jar in the fridge to chill, preferably for at least three hours.

4. Strain the water before serving.

Cucumber Lime with Basil and Mint

Ingredients:

- ½ cucumber, thinly sliced
- 1 lemon, thinly sliced
- ¼ cup fresh basil leaf, shredded
- 1/3 cup fresh mint leaves, shredded

Directions:

1. Put the cucumber and lemon slices into a two-quart glass jar or pitcher and press them lightly with a muddle or a wooden spoon, twisting the muddle enough to start releasing the juices. Don't pulverize the lemon or cucumber into pieces. Add the basil and mint.

2. If you plan to drink all or most of the fruit water within the next five hours, fill the jar halfway with ice and then top the jar off with cold drinking water. If you're planning to store the water for longer than five hours before drinking it, fill the jar three-quarters full of ice before topping it off with water.

3. Stir with a chopstick or long spoon and put a lid on the jar. Stick the jar in the fridge to chill, preferably for at least three hours.

4. Strain the water before serving.

Watermelon Lime and Basil

Ingredients:

- 2 cups of thin triangular wedges of watermelon, honeydew or cantaloupe

- 1 lime, sliced thinly

- 4 basil leaves, torn in half

Directions:

1. Put the basil into a one-quart glass jar and press them lightly with a muddle or a wooden spoon. Add the melon and lime and press them, twisting the muddle to start releasing the fruit juices. Don't pulverize the herbs or fruit into pieces.

2. If you plan to drink all or most of the fruit water within the next five hours, fill the jar halfway with ice and then top the jar off with cold drinking water. If you're planning to store the water for longer than five hours before drinking it, fill the jar three-quarters full of ice before topping it off with water.

3. Stir with a chopstick or long spoon and put a lid on the jar. Stick the jar in the fridge to chill, preferably for at least three hours.

4. Strain the water before serving.

Berry Spice

Ingredients:

- 2 cups raspberries or blackberries
- 1 orange or lime, cut in half and sliced thinly
- Borage flowers or leaves

Directions:

1. Put the borage into a one-quart glass jar and press it lightly with a muddle or a wooden spoon. Add the fruits and press them, twisting the muddle to start releasing the fruit juices. Don't pulverize the spices or fruit into pieces.

2. If you plan to drink all or most of the fruit water within the next five hours, fill the jar halfway with ice and then top the jar off with cold drinking water. If you're planning to store the water for longer than five hours before drinking it, fill the jar three-quarters full of ice before topping it off with water.

3. Stir with a chopstick or long spoon and put a lid on the jar. Stick the jar in the fridge to chill, preferably for at least three hours.

4. Strain the water before serving.

Rose Spice

Ingredients:

- ½ cup basil, preferably holy basil
- ½ cup rose petals
- Splash of organic rose water OR 1 drop of rose oil

Directions:

1. Put the basil into a one-quart glass jar and press it lightly with a muddle or a wooden spoon. Don't pulverize the basil into pieces. Add the rose petals.

2. If you plan to drink all or most of the fruit water within the next five hours, fill the jar halfway with ice and then top the jar off with cold drinking water. If you're planning to store the water for longer than five hours before drinking it, fill the jar three-quarters full of ice before topping it off with water.

3. Stir with a chopstick or long spoon and put a lid on the jar. Stick the jar in the fridge to chill, preferably for at least three hours.

4. Strain the water before serving.

Peach Vanilla

Ingredients:

- 2 peaches, pitted and sliced
- 1 vanilla bean, sliced lengthwise

Directions:

1. Put the peaches into a one-quart glass jar and press them with a muddle or a wooden spoon, twisting the muddle to start releasing the fruit juices. Don't pulverize the fruit into pieces.

2. Scrape the vanilla out of the bean and add it to the peaches. You can optionally also add the bean itself to the jar.

3. If you plan to drink all or most of the fruit water within the next five hours, fill the jar halfway with ice and then top the jar off with cold drinking water. If you're planning to store the water for longer than five hours before drinking it, fill the jar three-quarters full of ice before topping it off with water.

4. Stir with a chopstick or long spoon and put a lid on the jar. Stick the jar in the fridge to chill, preferably for at least three hours.

5. Strain the water before serving.

Cardamom, Vanilla and Orange

Ingredients:

- 1 orange, peeled and sliced
- 1 tbsp. cardamom
- 1 vanilla bean, sliced lengthwise

Directions:

1. Put the cardamom into a one-quart glass jar and press it lightly with a muddle or a wooden spoon. Add the orange slices and press them, twisting the muddle to start releasing the fruit juices. Don't pulverize the cardamom or orange slices into pieces.

2. Scrape the vanilla out of the bean and add it to the jar. You can optionally also add the bean itself to the jar.

3. If you plan to drink all or most of the fruit water within the next five hours, fill the jar halfway with ice and then top the jar off with cold drinking water. If you're planning to store the water for longer than five hours before drinking it, fill the jar three-quarters full of ice before topping it off with water.

4. Stir with a chopstick or long spoon and put a lid on the jar. Stick the jar in the fridge to chill, preferably for at least three hours.

5. Strain the water before serving.

Watermelon-Jalapeno Cooler

Ingredients:

- 1 jalapeno, stemmed, seeded
- 4 sprigs fresh thyme
- 10 cups watermelon, seeded, chopped
- 1 cup hot water
- 8 cups filtered water

Directions:

1. Add jalapeno and thyme to hot water. Let it infuse for 5 minutes. Discard the jalapeno and thyme and pour into the glass jar.

2. Add the water melon and press, twisting the muddle to start releasing the fruit juices. Don't pulverize the water melon into pieces.

3. If you plan to drink all or most of the fruit water within the next five hours, fill the jar halfway with ice and then top the jar off with cold drinking water. If you're planning to store the water for longer than five hours before drinking it, fill the jar three-quarters full of ice before topping it off with water.

4. Stir with a chopstick or long spoon and put a lid on the jar. Stick the jar in the fridge to chill, preferably for at least three hours.

5. Strain the water before serving.

Mango Ginger Delight

Ingredients:

- 2 inch piece fresh ginger root, peeled, sliced
- 2 cups ripe mango pieces
- 6 cups ice
- 6 cups water

Directions:

1. Add all the ingredients to a glass jar. Stir well. Fasten the lid.

2. Refrigerate for 4-5 hours. Strain and serve the infused water.

Raspberry, Rose Petal, and Vanilla

Ingredients:

- 2 cups raspberries
- 1 cup rose petals
- 1 pod vanilla, cut lengthwise

Directions:

1. Put the raspberries into a large glass jar and press them with a muddle or a wooden spoon, twisting the muddle to start releasing the fruit juices. Don't pulverize the fruit into pieces.

2. Scrape the vanilla out of the bean and add it to the raspberries. You can optionally also add the bean itself to the jar.

3. If you plan to drink all or most of the fruit water within the next five hours, fill the jar halfway with ice and then top the jar off with cold drinking water. If you're planning to store the water for longer than five hours

before drinking it, fill the jar three-quarters full of ice before topping it off with water.

4. Stir with a chopstick or long spoon and put a lid on the jar. Stick the jar in the fridge to chill, preferably for at least three hours.

5. Strain the water before serving.

Spicy Orange Water

Ingredients:

- 2 oranges, peeled, seeded, sliced into segments
- 2 pods cardamom
- 4-5 cloves
- 1 inch stick cinnamon
- 1 teaspoon allspice

Directions:

1. Put the, cinnamon, cloves, allspice and cardamom into a one-quart glass jar and press it lightly with a muddle or a wooden spoon. Add the orange slices and press them, twisting the muddle to start releasing the fruit juices. Don't pulverize the cardamom or orange slices into pieces.

2. If you plan to drink all or most of the fruit water within the next five hours, fill the jar halfway with ice and then

top the jar off with cold drinking water. If you're planning to store the water for longer than five hours before drinking it, fill the jar three-quarters full of ice before topping it off with water.

3. Stir with a chopstick or long spoon and put a lid on the jar. Stick the jar in the fridge to chill, preferably for at least three hours.

4. Strain the water before serving.

Fennel & Curry Leaves

Ingredients:

- 1 cup curry leaves, torn
- 2 fennel bulbs, thinly sliced (white as well as green parts)
- 6 glasses water

Directions:

1. Add all the ingredients to a glass jar. Stir well. Fasten the lid.
2. Refrigerate for 4-5 hours. Strain and serve the infused water.

Turmeric Ginger Tangerine

Ingredients:

- 1 small piece of ginger
- 1 tangerine, peeled and sliced
- 2 inch piece fresh turmeric

Directions:

1. Skin the ginger and turmeric and slice it into small rings. Put it into a one-quart glass jar and press it lightly with a muddle or a wooden spoon. Add the tangerine slices and press them, twisting them enough to start releasing the fruit juices. Don't pulverize the herbs or fruit into pieces.

2. If you plan to drink all or most of the fruit water within the next five hours, fill the jar halfway with ice and then top the jar off with cold drinking water. If you're planning to store the water for longer than five hours before drinking it, fill the jar three-quarters full of ice before topping it off with water.

3. Stir with a chopstick or long spoon and put a lid on the jar. Stick the jar in the fridge to chill, preferably for at least three hours.

4. Strain the water before serving.

Spicy Concoction

Ingredients:

- 2 pods green cardamom
- 1 inch piece ginger, peeled, sliced
- 8-10 black pepper
- ½ a jalapeno pepper, sliced
- 1 cucumber, sliced
- 10 strawberries, sliced

Directions:

1. Put the ginger, pepper, and cardamom into a 2-quart glass jar and press it lightly with a muddle or a wooden spoon. Add the strawberry and cucumber slices and press them, twisting the muddle to start releasing the fruit juices. Add the jalapeno .Don't pulverize the spices into pieces.

2. If you plan to drink all or most of the fruit water within the next five hours, fill the jar halfway with ice and then top the jar off with cold drinking water. If you're planning to store the water for longer than five hours before drinking it, fill the jar three-quarters full of ice before topping it off with water.

3. Stir with a chopstick or long spoon and put a lid on the jar. Stick the jar in the fridge to chill, preferably for at least three hours.

4. Strain the water before serving.

Chapter 5.
Herb Recipes

These recipes include one or more herbs, in addition to fruit and sometimes a vegetable. Feel free to get creative here, substituting ingredients according to your taste.

Basil, Cucumber and Lime

Ingredients:

- 1 sprig fresh basil
- 6 slices cucumber
- 2 slices lime

Directions:

1. Put the basil into a one-quart glass jar and press it lightly with a muddle or a wooden spoon. Add the lime and cucumber, pressing and twisting them enough to start releasing the fruit juices. Don't pulverize the basil or fruit into pieces.

2. If you plan to drink all or most of the fruit water within the next five hours, fill the jar halfway with ice and then top the jar off with cold drinking water. If you're planning to store the water for longer than five hours before drinking it, fill the jar three-quarters full of ice before topping it off with water.

3. Stir with a chopstick or long spoon and put a lid on the jar. Stick the jar in the fridge to chill, preferably for at least three hours.

4. Strain the water before serving.

Rosemary and Friends

Ingredients:

- 1 sprig fresh rosemary
- 1 lemon, sliced
- 1 peach, sliced
- 1 handful raspberries

Directions:

1. Put the rosemary into a two-quart glass jar or pitcher and press it lightly with a muddle or a wooden spoon. Rosemary has a strong flavor, so it barely needs to be pressed. Add the fruits and press them also, twisting them enough to start releasing the fruit juices. Don't pulverize the herbs or fruit into pieces.

2. If you plan to drink all or most of the fruit water within the next five hours, fill the jar halfway with ice and then top the jar off with cold drinking water. If you're planning to store the water for longer than five hours before drinking it, fill the jar three-quarters full of ice before topping it off with water.

3. Stir with a chopstick or long spoon and put a lid on the jar. Stick the jar in the fridge to chill, preferably for at least three hours.

4. Strain the water before serving.

Mint and Cucumber

Ingredients:

- 1/2 cucumber, sliced
- 10 mint leaves, torn in half

Directions:

1. Put the mint into a two-quart glass jar and press it lightly with a muddle or a wooden spoon. Add the cucumber slices and press them, twisting them enough to start releasing the juice. Don't pulverize the mint or cucumber into pieces.

2. If you plan to drink all or most of the fruit water within the next five hours, fill the jar halfway with ice and then top the jar off with cold drinking water. If you're planning to store the water for longer than five hours before drinking it, fill the jar three-quarters full of ice before topping it off with water.

3. Stir with a chopstick or long spoon and put a lid on the jar. Stick the jar in the fridge to chill, preferably for at least three hours.

4. Strain the water before serving.

Blackberry and Sage

Ingredients:

- 1 cup blackberries
- 4 sage leaves

Directions:

1. Tear the sage leaves in half and put them into a two-quart glass jar or pitcher and press them lightly with a muddle or a wooden spoon. Add the blackberries and press them also, twisting them enough to start releasing the fruit juices. Don't pulverize the sage or blackberries into pieces.

2. If you plan to drink all or most of the fruit water within the next five hours, fill the jar halfway with ice and then top the jar off with cold drinking water. If you're planning to store the water for longer than five hours before drinking it, fill the jar three-quarters full of ice before topping it off with water.

3. Stir with a chopstick or long spoon and put a lid on the jar. Stick the jar in the fridge to chill, preferably for at least three hours.

4. Strain the water before serving.

Rosemary and Watermelon

Ingredients:

- 2 fresh rosemary stems
- 1 cup of watermelon, cut into cubes

Directions:

1. Put the rosemary into a two-quart glass jar or pitcher and press it lightly with a muddle or a wooden spoon. Add the watermelon cubes and press them also, twisting them enough to start releasing the fruit juices. Don't pulverize the rosemary or watermelon into pieces.

2. If you plan to drink all or most of the fruit water within the next five hours, fill the jar halfway with ice and then top the jar off with cold drinking water. If you're planning to store the water for longer than five hours before drinking it, fill the jar three-quarters full of ice before topping it off with water.

3. Stir with a chopstick or long spoon and put a lid on the jar. Stick the jar in the fridge to chill, preferably for at least three hours.

4. Strain the water before serving.

Mint, Basil, Lime and Cucumber

Ingredients:

- ¼ cup fresh basil, finely chopped

- 1/3 cup fresh mint, finely chopped

- 1 cucumber

- 1 lemon

Directions:

1. Put the mint and basil into a two-quart glass jar or pitcher and press them lightly with a muddle or a wooden spoon. Add the cucumber and lemon, pressing and twisting them enough to start releasing the fruit juices. Don't pulverize the herbs or fruit into pieces.

2. If you plan to drink all or most of the fruit water within the next five hours, fill the jar halfway with ice and then top the jar off with cold drinking water. If you're planning to store the water for longer than five hours before drinking it, fill the jar three-quarters full of ice before topping it off with water.

3. Stir with a chopstick or long spoon and put a lid on the jar. Stick the jar in the fridge to chill, preferably for at least three hours.

4. Strain the water before serving.

Rosemary, Orange and Lime

Ingredients:

- 1 sprig of rosemary

- 2 slices of lime

- 1 slice of orange

Directions:

1. Put the rosemary into a one-quart glass jar and press it lightly with a muddle or a wooden spoon. Add the lime and orange slices and press them, twisting them enough to start releasing the fruit juices. Don't pulverize the herbs or fruit into pieces.

2. If you plan to drink all or most of the fruit water within the next five hours, fill the jar halfway with ice and then top the jar off with cold drinking water. If you're planning to store the water for longer than five hours before drinking it, fill the jar three-quarters full of ice before topping it off with water.

3. Stir with a chopstick or long spoon and put a lid on the jar. Stick the jar in the fridge to chill, preferably for at least three hours.

4. Strain the water before serving.

Orange Lavender

Ingredients:

- 1 orange, peeled and sliced
- 2 sprigs lavender

Directions:

1. Put the lavender into a one-quart glass jar and press it lightly with a muddle or a wooden spoon. Add the orange slices and press them, twisting the muddle to start releasing the fruit juices. Don't pulverize the lavender or orange slices.

2. If you plan to drink all or most of the fruit water within the next five hours, fill the jar halfway with ice and then top the jar off with cold drinking water. If you're planning to store the water for longer than five hours before drinking it, fill the jar three-quarters full of ice before topping it off with water.

3. Stir with a chopstick or long spoon and put a lid on the jar. Stick the jar in the fridge to chill, preferably for at least three hours.

4. Strain the water before serving.

Mint, Plum, Apples and Blueberries

Ingredients:

- 4 mint leaves, finely chopped
- ½ apple, cored and sliced
- 1 plum, pit removed and sliced
- Handful of blueberries

Directions:

1. Put the mint into a one-quart glass jar and press it lightly with a muddle or a wooden spoon. Add all the fruit and muddle it just enough to start releasing the juices. Don't pulverize the mint or fruit into pieces.

2. If you plan to drink all or most of the fruit water within the next five hours, fill the jar halfway with ice and then top the jar off with cold drinking water. If you're planning to store the water for longer than five hours before drinking it, fill the jar three-quarters full of ice before topping it off with water.

3. Stir with a chopstick or long spoon and put a lid on the jar. Stick the jar in the fridge to chill, preferably for at least three hours.

4. Strain the water before serving.

Sage Honeydew

Ingredients:

- 4 sage leaves
- 5 pieces honeydew

Directions:

1. Put the sage into a one-quart glass jar and press it lightly with a muddle or a wooden spoon. Add the honeydew and muddle it just enough to start releasing the juices. Don't pulverize the sage or honeydew.

2. If you plan to drink all or most of the fruit water within the next five hours, fill the jar halfway with ice and then top the jar off with cold drinking water. If you're planning to store the water for longer than five hours before drinking it, fill the jar three-quarters full of ice before topping it off with water.

3. Stir with a chopstick or long spoon and put a lid on the jar. Stick the jar in the fridge to chill, preferably for at least three hours.

4. Strain the water before serving.

Sage Berry

Ingredients:

- 2 sage leaves
- 10 blackberries
- 10 raspberries

Directions:

1. Put the sage into a one-quart glass jar and press it lightly with a muddle or a wooden spoon. Add all the fruit and muddle it just enough to start releasing the juices, but not enough to mash it.

2. If you plan to drink all or most of the fruit water within the next five hours, fill the jar halfway with ice and then top the jar off with cold drinking water. If you're planning to store the water for longer than five hours

before drinking it, fill the jar three-quarters full of ice before topping it off with water.

3. Stir with a chopstick or long spoon and put a lid on the jar. Stick the jar in the fridge to chill, preferably for at least three hours.

4. Strain the water before serving.

Nutmeg Cranapple

Ingredients:

- ½ cup cranberries (fresh or frozen)
- 1 apple, thinly sliced
- ¼ lemon, sliced
- 1 pinch of ground nutmeg

Directions:

1. Put the cranberry and lemon into a one-quart glass jar and muddle them just enough to start releasing the juices, but not enough to mash them. Add the apple slices without muddling them. Toss the nutmeg into the jar.

2. If you plan to drink all or most of the fruit water within the next five hours, fill the jar halfway with ice and then top the jar off with cold drinking water. If you're planning to store the water for longer than five hours

before drinking it, fill the jar three-quarters full of ice before topping it off with water.

3. Stir with a chopstick or long spoon and put a lid on the jar. Stick the jar in the fridge to chill, preferably for at least three hours.

4. Strain the water before serving.

Lavender Kiwi

Ingredients:

- 1/8 cup lavender

- 2 kiwis, peeled and sliced

Directions:

1. Put the lavender into a one-quart glass jar and press it lightly with a muddle or a wooden spoon. Add the kiwi and muddle it just enough to start releasing the juices, but not enough to mash it.

2. If you plan to drink all or most of the fruit water within the next five hours, fill the jar halfway with ice and then top the jar off with cold drinking water. If you're planning to store the water for longer than five hours before drinking it, fill the jar three-quarters full of ice before topping it off with water.

3. Stir with a chopstick or long spoon and put a lid on the jar. Stick the jar in the fridge to chill, preferably for at least three hours.

4. Strain the water before serving.

Cinnamon Apple

Ingredients:

- 1 cinnamon stick
- ½ red apple, thinly sliced

Directions:

1. Put the apple and cinnamon into a two-quart glass jar or pitcher. Don't use ground cinnamon, because it will float.

2. If you plan to drink all or most of the fruit water within the next five hours, fill the jar half way with ice and then top the jar off with cold drinking water. If you're planning to store the water for longer than five hours before drinking it, fill the jar three-quarters full of ice before topping it off with water.

3. Stir with a chopstick or long spoon and put a lid on the jar. Stick the jar in the fridge to chill, preferably for at least three hours.

4. Strain the water before serving.

Pineapple Thyme

Ingredients:

- 5 sprigs of thyme

- ½ cup pineapple chunks

Directions:

1. Tear the thyme sprigs and put them into a one-quart glass jar. Add the pineapple and muddle it just enough to start releasing the juices, but not enough to mash it.

2. If you plan to drink all or most of the fruit water within the next five hours, fill the jar half way with ice and then top the jar off with cold drinking water. If you're planning to store the water for longer than five hours before drinking it, fill the jar three-quarters full of ice before topping it off with water.

3. Stir with a chopstick or long spoon and put a lid on the jar. Stick the jar in the fridge to chill, preferably for at least three hours.

4. Strain the water before serving.

Cranberry, Orange and Mint

Ingredients:

- 4 mint leaves

- ½ cup cranberries, fresh or frozen

- 1 orange, peeled and sliced

Directions:

1. Put the mint into a one-quart glass jar and press it lightly with a muddle or a wooden spoon. Add all the fruit and muddle it just enough to start releasing the juices, but not enough to mash it.

2. If you plan to drink all or most of the fruit water within the next five hours, fill the jar half way with ice and then top the jar off with cold drinking water. If you're planning to store the water for longer than five hours before drinking it, fill the jar three-quarters full of ice before topping it off with water.

3. Stir with a chopstick or long spoon and put a lid on the jar. Stick the jar in the fridge to chill, preferably for at least three hours.

4. Strain the water before serving.

Grapefruit, Sage and Strawberries

Ingredients:

- 2 sage leaves

- 1 cup strawberries, topped and sliced

- ½ grapefruit, peeled and sliced

Directions:

1. Tear the sage leaves and put them into a one-quart glass jar. Press the leaves lightly with a muddle or a wooden spoon. Add all the fruit and muddle it just enough to start releasing the juices, but not enough to mash it.

2. If you plan to drink all or most of the fruit water within the next five hours, fill the jar half way with ice and then top the jar off with cold drinking water. If you're planning to store the water for longer than five hours before drinking it, fill the jar three-quarters full of ice before topping it off with water.

3. Stir with a chopstick or long spoon and put a lid on the jar. Stick the jar in the fridge to chill, preferably for at least three hours.

4. Strain the water before serving.

Rosy Cukes

Ingredients:

- 2 sprigs rosemary
- 15 slices cucumber
- ½ grapefruit, peeled and sliced

Directions:

1. Put the rosemary into a one-quart glass jar and press it lightly with a muddle or a wooden spoon. Add the cucumber and grapefruit, and muddle them just enough to start releasing the juices, but not enough to mash it.

2. If you plan to drink all or most of the fruit water within the next five hours, fill the jar half way with ice and then top the jar off with cold drinking water. If you're planning to store the water for longer than five hours before drinking it, fill the jar three-quarters full of ice before topping it off with water.

3. Stir with a chopstick or long spoon and put a lid on the jar. Stick the jar in the fridge to chill, preferably for at least three hours.

4. Strain the water before serving.

Blueberry, Orange and Basil

Ingredients:

- 6 basil leaves
- 10 blueberries
- 2 slices orange

Directions:

1. Tear the basil leaves and put them into a one-quart glass jar. Press them lightly with a muddle or a wooden

spoon. Add the blueberries and oranges, and muddle them just enough to start releasing the juices, but not enough to mash them.

2. If you plan to drink all or most of the fruit water within the next five hours, fill the jar half way with ice and then top the jar off with cold drinking water. If you're planning to store the water for longer than five hours before drinking it, fill the jar three-quarters full of ice before topping it off with water.

3. Stir with a chopstick or long spoon and put a lid on the jar. Stick the jar in the fridge to chill, preferably for at least three hours.

4. Strain the water before serving.

Basil Mango

Ingredients:

- 8 basil leaves
- 1 ripe mango; cored, peeled and cubed

Directions:

1. Tear the basil leaves and put them into a one-quart glass jar. Press them lightly with a muddle or a wooden spoon. Add the mango and muddle it just enough to start releasing the juices, but not enough to mash it.

2. If you plan to drink all or most of the fruit water within the next five hours, fill the jar half way with ice and

then top the jar off with cold drinking water. If you're planning to store the water for longer than five hours before drinking it, fill the jar three-quarters full of ice before topping it off with water.

3. Stir with a chopstick or long spoon and put a lid on the jar. Stick the jar in the fridge to chill, preferably for at least three hours.

4. Strain the water before serving.

Strawberry Cucumber Basil

Ingredients:

- 6-7 basil leaves roughly chopped
- 2 strawberries; sliced
- 8-10 slices cucumber
- Ice
- 2 glasses water

Directions:

1. Add all the ingredients to a glass jar. Close the lid. Let it infuse at least for an hour at room temperature.
2. Strain and serve the water.

Lemongrass Mint

Ingredients:

- 4 pieces lemongrass (each about 2 inches)
- 15-20 mint leaves, torn
- 8 glasses water

Directions:

1. Add all the ingredients to a glass jar. Stir well. Fasten the lid.
2. Refrigerate for 4-5 hours. Strain and serve the infused water.

Pineapple-Strawberry Cooler

Ingredients:

- ½ cup strawberries
- ½ cup pineapple
- 2 sage leaves
- 8 glasses water

Directions:

1. Add all the ingredients to a glass jar. Stir well. Fasten the lid.

2. Refrigerate for 4-5 hours. Strain and serve the infused water.

Rosemary and Grapefruit

Ingredients:

- 1 grapefruit, peeled, cut into segments
- Lots of sprigs of rosemary (more the better)
- 8-10 glasses water

Directions:

1. Add all the ingredients to a glass jar. Stir well. Fasten the lid.
2. Refrigerate for 7-8 hours. Strain and serve the infused water.

True Blue

Ingredients:

- 2 ½ cups blueberries
- Lavender flowers (edible parts only)
- 10 cups water

Directions:

1. Add all the ingredients to a glass jar. Stir well. Fasten the lid.

2. Refrigerate for 4-5 hours. Strain and serve the infused water.

Vanilla Basil Strawberry

Ingredients:

- 1 cup strawberries, sliced
- 1 vanilla pod, cut lengthwise
- 10-12 leaves fresh basil

Directions:

1. Put the strawberries into a one-quart glass jar and press them with a muddle or a wooden spoon, twisting the muddle to start releasing the fruit juices. Don't pulverize the strawberries into pieces.

2. Scrape the vanilla out of the bean and add it to the jar. You can optionally also add the bean itself to the jar. Add the basil leaves.

3. If you plan to drink all or most of the fruit water within the next five hours, fill the jar halfway with ice and then top the jar off with cold drinking water. If you're planning to store the water for longer than five hours

before drinking it, fill the jar three-quarters full of ice before topping it off with water.

4. Stir with a chopstick or long spoon and put a lid on the jar. Stick the jar in the fridge to chill, preferably for at least three hours.

5. Strain the water before serving.

Fennel & Pear

Ingredients:

- 1 ripe and firm pear, peeled, seeded, sliced
- 2 fennel bulbs, thinly sliced (white as well as green parts)
- 6 glasses water

Directions:

1. Add all the ingredients to a glass jar. Stir well. Fasten the lid.
2. Refrigerate for 4-5 hours. Strain and serve the infused water.

Blueberry Cucumber & Basil

Ingredients:

- 1 cup fresh blueberries

- 6-7 slices cucumber
- 10-12 basil leaves

Directions:

1. Put the basil into a two-quart glass jar or pitcher and press them lightly with a muddle or a wooden spoon. Add the cucumber and blueberries, pressing and twisting them enough to start releasing the fruit juices. Don't pulverize the blueberries or cucumber into pieces.

2. If you plan to drink all or most of the fruit water within the next five hours, fill the jar halfway with ice and then top the jar off with cold drinking water. If you're planning to store the water for longer than five hours before drinking it, fill the jar three-quarters full of ice before topping it off with water.

3. Stir with a chopstick or long spoon and put a lid on the jar. Stick the jar in the fridge to chill, preferably for at least three hours.

4. Strain the water before serving.

Orange Lavender

Ingredients:

- 1 lemon, peeled and sliced
- 3-4 sprigs lavender

Directions:

1. Put the lavender into a one-quart glass jar and press it lightly with a muddle or a wooden spoon. Add the lemon slices and press them, twisting the muddle to start releasing the fruit juices. Don't pulverize the lavender or lemon slices.

2. If you plan to drink all or most of the fruit water within the next five hours, fill the jar halfway with ice and then top the jar off with cold drinking water. If you're planning to store the water for longer than five hours before drinking it, fill the jar three-quarters full of ice before topping it off with water.

3. Stir with a chopstick or long spoon and put a lid on the jar. Stick the jar in the fridge to chill, preferably for at least three hours.

4. Strain the water before serving.

Raspberry & Rose

Ingredients:

1 cup raspberries

1 cup fresh rose petals

2 teaspoons organic rose water

6 cups water

Directions:

Add all the ingredients to a glass jar. Stir well. Fasten the lid. Refrigerate for 4-5 hours. Strain and serve the infused water.

Mango Pineapple Mint

- 1 cup pineapple chunks
- ½ cup mango chunks
- ½ cup mint leaves, torn

Directions:

1. Put all the mint, pineapple and mango chunks into a one-quart glass jar and press it with a wooden spoon or muddle, twisting it slightly until the fruit begins to release its juices. Don't pulverize the fruit into pieces.

2. Fill the glass jar with the water. If you plan to drink all or most of the fruit water within the next five hours, fill the jar halfway with ice and then top the jar off with cold drinking water.

3. Stir with a chopstick or long spoon and put a lid on the jar. Stick the jar in the fridge to chill, preferably for at least three hours.

4. Strain the water before serving.

Chapter 6. Minced Herb Recipes

These recipes call for minced herbs, so the herbs release their flavor more quickly than herbs that have only been muddled. This allows you to use a smaller quantity if you want, and you don't have to let them soak as long. But it also means you'll probably only be able to use these herbs for one or possibly two batches.

Citrus, Basil and Mint

Ingredients:

- 1 lime, sliced
- 1 lemon, sliced
- 1 small grapefruit, sliced
- 1 small orange, sliced
- 2 tablespoons minced mint
- 2 tablespoons minced basil

Directions:

1. Put the fruit slices into a two-quart jar or pitcher and press them, twisting them enough to start releasing the fruit juices. Don't pulverize the fruit into pieces. Mince the herbs finely and add them to the mixture.

2. If you plan to drink all or most of the fruit water within the next five hours, fill the jar halfway with ice and then

top the jar off with cold drinking water. If you're planning to store the water for longer than five hours before drinking it, fill the jar three-quarters full of ice before topping it off with water.

3. Stir with a chopstick or long spoon and put a lid on the jar. Stick the jar in the fridge to chill, preferably for at least three hours.

4. Strain the water before serving.

Mint, Cucumber and Lemon

Ingredients:

- 1 small cucumber, sliced
- 1 lemon, sliced
- 2 tablespoons minced mint

Directions:

1. Put the lemon and cucumber slices into a two-quart jar or pitcher and press them, twisting them enough to start releasing the juices. Don't pulverize them into pieces. Mince the mint finely and add it to the mixture.

2. If you plan to drink all or most of the fruit water within the next five hours, fill the jar halfway with ice and then top the jar off with cold drinking water. If you're planning to store the water for longer than five hours before drinking it, fill the jar three-quarters full of ice before topping it off with water.

3. Stir with a chopstick or long spoon and put a lid on the jar. Stick the jar in the fridge to chill, preferably for at least three hours.

4. Strain the water before serving.

Berry and Sage

Ingredients:

- 1 cup whole berries (blackberries, raspberries, blueberries, or a mix)
- 1 tablespoon minced sage

Directions:

1. Put the berries into a two-quart jar or pitcher and press them, twisting them enough to start releasing the juices. Don't pulverize them into pieces. Mince the sage finely and add it to the mixture.

2. If you plan to drink all or most of the fruit water within the next five hours, fill the jar halfway with ice and then top the jar off with cold drinking water. If you're planning to store the water for longer than five hours before drinking it, fill the jar three-quarters full of ice before topping it off with water.

3. Stir with a chopstick or long spoon and put a lid on the jar. Stick the jar in the fridge to chill, preferably for at least three hours.

4. Strain the water before serving.

Mint Pineapple

Ingredients:

- 1 cup cubed pineapple
- 2 tablespoons minced mint

Directions:

1. Put the pineapple cubes into a two-quart jar or pitcher and press them, twisting them enough to start releasing the juices. Don't pulverize them into pieces. Mince the mint finely and add it to the mixture.

2. If you plan to drink all or most of the fruit water within the next five hours, fill the jar halfway with ice and then top the jar off with cold drinking water. If you're planning to store the water for longer than five hours before drinking it, fill the jar three-quarters full of ice before topping it off with water.

3. Stir with a chopstick or long spoon and put a lid on the jar. Stick the jar in the fridge to chill, preferably for at least three hours.

4. Strain the water before serving.

Basil, Kiwi and Strawberry

Ingredients:

- 1 cup halved strawberries

- 1 cup cubed kiwi (or use 1 lime, sliced)
- 2 tablespoons minced basil

Directions:

1. Put the strawberries and kiwi into a two-quart jar or pitcher and press them, twisting them enough to start releasing the juices. Don't pulverize them into pieces. Mince the basil finely and add to the mixture.

2. If you plan to drink all or most of the fruit water within the next five hours, fill the jar halfway with ice and then top the jar off with cold drinking water. If you're planning to store the water for longer than five hours before drinking it, fill the jar three-quarters full of ice before topping it off with water.

3. Stir with a chopstick or long spoon and put a lid on the jar. Stick the jar in the fridge to chill, preferably for at least three hours.

4. Strain the water before serving.

Rosemary, Grapefruit and Orange

Ingredients:

- 1 small grapefruit, sliced
- 1 small orange, sliced
- 1 tablespoon minced rosemary

Directions:

1. Put the orange and grapefruit slices into a two-quart jar or pitcher and press them, twisting them enough to start releasing the juices. Don't pulverize them into pieces. Mince the rosemary finely and add it to the mixture.

2. If you plan to drink all or most of the fruit water within the next five hours, fill the jar halfway with ice and then top the jar off with cold drinking water. If you're planning to store the water for longer than five hours before drinking it, fill the jar three-quarters full of ice before topping it off with water.

3. Stir with a chopstick or long spoon and put a lid on the jar. Stick the jar in the fridge to chill, preferably for at least three hours.

4. Strain the water before serving.

Mint, Lime and Watermelon

Ingredients:

- 1 cup cubed watermelon
- 1 lime, sliced
- 2 tablespoons minced mint

Directions:

1. Put the watermelon and lime into a two-quart jar or pitcher and press them, twisting them enough to start releasing the juices. Don't pulverize them into pieces. Mince the mint finely and add it to the mixture.

2. If you plan to drink all or most of the fruit water within the next five hours, fill the jar halfway with ice and then top the jar off with cold drinking water. If you're planning to store the water for longer than five hours before drinking it, fill the jar three-quarters full of ice before topping it off with water.

3. Stir with a chopstick or long spoon and put a lid on the jar. Stick the jar in the fridge to chill, preferably for at least three hours.

4. Strain the water before serving.

Tarragon, Lime and Cherry

Ingredients:

- 1 cup pitted and halved cherries

- 1 lime, sliced

- 1 tablespoon minced tarragon (or use 2 tablespoons minced mint)

Directions:

1. Put the cherries and lime into a two-quart jar or pitcher and press them, twisting them enough to start releasing the juices. Don't pulverize them into pieces. Mince the tarragon or mint finely and add it to the mixture.

2. If you plan to drink all or most of the fruit water within the next five hours, fill the jar halfway with ice and then top the jar off with cold drinking water. If you're planning to store the water for longer than five hours before drinking it, fill the jar three-quarters full of ice before topping it off with water.

3. Stir with a chopstick or long spoon and put a lid on the jar. Stick the jar in the fridge to chill, preferably for at least three hours.

4. Strain the water before serving.

Thyme, Peach and Blueberry

Ingredients:

- 1 cup whole blueberries
- 1 cup cubed peaches
- 1 tablespoon minced thyme

Directions:

1. Put the blueberries and peaches into a two-quart jar or pitcher and press them, twisting them enough to start

releasing the juices. Don't pulverize them into pieces. Take your thyme and mince it finely, then add it to the mixture.

2. If you plan to drink all or most of the fruit water within the next five hours, fill the jar halfway with ice and then top the jar off with cold drinking water. If you're planning to store the water for longer than five hours before drinking it, fill the jar three-quarters full of ice before topping it off with water.

3. Stir with a chopstick or long spoon and put a lid on the jar. Stick the jar in the fridge to chill, preferably for at least three hours.

4. Strain the water before serving.

Mint Peach

Ingredients:

- 1 cup cubed peaches
- 2 tablespoons minced mint

Directions:

1. Put the peaches into a two-quart jar or pitcher and press them, twisting them enough to start releasing the juices. Don't pulverize them into pieces. Mince the mint finely and add it to the mixture.

2. If you plan to drink all or most of the fruit water within the next five hours, fill the jar halfway with ice and then

top the jar off with cold drinking water. If you're planning to store the water for longer than five hours before drinking it, fill the jar three-quarters full of ice before topping it off with water.

3. Stir with a chopstick or long spoon and put a lid on the jar. Stick the jar in the fridge to chill, preferably for at least three hours.

4. Strain the water before serving.

Tropical Mince herbed water

Ingredients:

- 1 cup chopped pineapple
- 1 cup chopped mangoes
- 1 bunch cilantro, minced
- 3 cups coconut water
- 3 cups filtered water

Directions:

1. Add all the ingredients to a glass jar. Stir well. Fasten the lid.

2. Refrigerate for 1-2 hours. Strain and serve the infused water.

Green apple Raspberry Rosemary

Ingredients:

- 1 green apple, cored, sliced
- 1 cup raspberries
- 2 tablespoons minced rosemary

Directions:

1. Put the apple slices and rosemary into a two-quart jar or pitcher and press them, twisting them enough to start releasing the juices. Don't pulverize them into pieces. Add the rosemary.

2. If you plan to drink all or most of the fruit water within the next five hours, fill the jar halfway with ice and then top the jar off with cold drinking water. If you're planning to store the water for longer than five hours before drinking it, fill the jar three-quarters full of ice before topping it off with water.

3. Stir with a chopstick or long spoon and put a lid on the jar. Stick the jar in the fridge to chill, preferably for at least three hours.

4. Strain the water before serving.

Kiwi Blackberry Thyme & Basil

Ingredients:

- 1 kiwi, peeled, sliced
- 1 cup blackberries
- 1 tablespoon minced basil
- ½ tablespoon minced thyme

Directions:

1. Put the kiwi and blackberries into a two-quart jar or pitcher and press them, twisting them enough to start releasing the juices. Don't pulverize them into pieces. Add basil and thyme to the mixture.

2. If you plan to drink all or most of the fruit water within the next five hours, fill the jar halfway with ice and then top the jar off with cold drinking water. If you're planning to store the water for longer than five hours before drinking it, fill the jar three-quarters full of ice before topping it off with water.

3. Stir with a chopstick or long spoon and put a lid on the jar. Stick the jar in the fridge to chill, preferably for at least three hours.

4. Strain the water before serving

Root Delight

Ingredients:

- 1 small beetroot, peeled, sliced and the greens minced
- 1 carrot, peeled, sliced and the greens minced
- 2 inch piece fresh turmeric, sliced
- ¼ cup minced garlic greens
- 10 cups water

Directions:

1. Add all the ingredients to a glass jar. Stir well. Fasten the lid.
2. Refrigerate for 3-4 hours. Strain and serve the infused water.

Black Lady

Ingredients:

- 1 cup black grapes
- 1 cup blackberries
- ½ cup lavender flowers
- 2 tablespoons minced mint
- 8 cups water

Directions:

1. Add all the ingredients to a glass jar. Stir well. Fasten the lid.

2. Refrigerate for 1-2 hours. Strain and serve the infused water.

Carrot Cooler

Ingredients:

- 1 large carrot, peeled, sliced
- 1 small cucumber sliced
- 1 tablespoon minced celery
- 1 tablespoon minced parsley
- 6 cups water

Directions:

1. Add all the ingredients to a glass jar. Stir well. Fasten the lid.

2. Refrigerate for 1-2 hours. Strain and serve the infused water.

Chapter 7.
More Recipes

Here are a few change-of-pace recipes for a little more variety.

Cucumber Citrus

Ingredients:

- ½ grapefruit, peeled and sliced
- ½ blood orange, peeled and sliced
- ½ cucumber, sliced

Directions:

1. Put the cucumber and fruit into a one-quart glass jar or pitcher and press it with a wooden spoon or muddler, twisting it slightly until the fruit begins to release its juices. Don't pulverize the fruit into pieces.

2. If you plan to drink all or most of the fruit water within the next five hours, fill the jar halfway with ice and then top the jar off with cold drinking water. If you're planning to store the water for longer than five hours before drinking it, fill the jar three-quarters full of ice before topping it off with water.

3. Stir with a chopstick or long spoon and put a lid on the jar. Stick the jar in the fridge to chill, preferably for at least three hours.

4. Strain the water before serving.

Pineapple Cucumber

Ingredients:

- ½ cup pineapple, cut into chunks
- 1/3 cucumber, sliced into rings

Directions:

1. Put the pineapple and cucumber into a one-quart glass jar and press them with a wooden spoon or muddler, twisting it slightly until the fruit begins to release its juices. Don't pulverize the fruit into pieces.

2. If you plan to drink all or most of the fruit water within the next five hours, fill the jar halfway with ice and then top the jar off with cold drinking water. If you're planning to store the water for longer than five hours before drinking it, fill the jar three-quarters full of ice before topping it off with water.

3. Stir with a chopstick or long spoon and put a lid on the jar. Stick the jar in the fridge to chill, preferably for at least three hours.

4. Strain the water before serving.

Strawberry Chamomile

Ingredients:

- 1 orange, sliced
- 10 strawberries (tops removed and sliced)
- 2 chamomile tea bags

Directions:

1. Bring a half quart of water to a boil and then remove it from heat. Put the tea bags into a jar and pour the hot water over them. Steep for ten minutes, then remove the tea bags and let the water cool.

2. Put the orange slices and strawberries into a separate one-quart jar. Press the orange slices strawberries with a muddle or wooden spoon until the juice starts to release from the fruit. Don't pulverize the fruit.

3. Pour the cooled tea into the jar of fruit and fill the jar with ice, topping it with water. Put a lid on the jar and stick it in the fridge for at least three hours before serving.

4. Strain the water before serving.

Cucumber Lemon

Ingredients:

- 5 slices cucumber

- 4 slices lemon, peeled, with seeds removed

Directions:

1. Put the fruit into a one-quart glass jar and press it with a wooden spoon or muddler, twisting it slightly until the fruit begins to release its juices. Don't pulverize the fruit into pieces.

2. If you plan to drink all or most of the fruit water within the next five hours, fill the jar halfway with ice and then top the jar off with cold drinking water. If you're planning to store the water for longer than five hours before drinking it, fill the jar three-quarters full of ice before topping it off with water.

3. Stir with a chopstick or long spoon and put a lid on the jar. Stick the jar in the fridge to chill, preferably for at least three hours.

4. Strain the water before serving.

Ginger Tea

Ingredients:

- 1 teaspoon ginger, cut into small cubes
- 2 cups of tea water (your choice)

Directions:

1. 2 cups of water to a boil and then remove it from heat. Put the tea bags and ginger into a jar and pour the hot

water over them. Steep for ten minutes, then remove the tea bags and let the water cool.

2. Pour the cooled tea into a two-quart glass jar or pitcher and fill the jar with ice, topping it off with cold water. Put a lid on the jar and stick it in the fridge for at least three hours.

3. Strain the water before serving.

Cucumber Melon

Ingredients:

- ½ medium cucumber, sliced
- ¼ cantaloupe, cubed
- ¼ honeydew melon, cubed

Directions:

1. Cut the melon from their rinds and cut the fruit into cubes. Slice the cucumber.

2. Put all the ingredients into a one-quart glass jar and press them with a wooden spoon or muddler, twisting the muddler slightly until the fruit begins to release its juices. Don't pulverize the fruit into pieces.

3. If you plan to drink all or most of the flavored water within the next five hours, fill the jar halfway with ice and then top the jar off with cold drinking water. If you're planning to store the water for longer than five

hours before drinking it, fill the jar three-quarters full of ice before topping it off with water.

4. Stir with a chopstick or long spoon and put a lid on the jar. Stick the jar in the fridge to chill, preferably for at least three hours.

5. Strain the water before serving.

Strawberry, Cucumber and Citrus

Ingredients:

- ½ lemon, sliced

- ½ lime, sliced

- ½ orange, sliced

- 1 handful strawberries, sliced

- 6 slices cucumber

Directions:

1. Put the fruit and cucumber into a one-quart glass jar and press it with a wooden spoon or muddler, twisting it slightly until the fruit begins to release its juices. Don't pulverize the fruit into pieces.

2. If you plan to drink all or most of the fruit water within the next five hours, fill the jar halfway with ice and then top the jar off with cold drinking water. If you're planning to store the water for longer than five hours

before drinking it, fill the jar three-quarters full of ice before topping it off with water.

3. Stir with a chopstick or long spoon and put a lid on the jar. Stick the jar in the fridge to chill, preferably for at least three hours.

4. Strain the water before serving.

Blood Orange

Ingredients:

- ½ grapefruit (peeled and sliced)
- ½ blood orange (peeled and sliced)
- ½ cucumber (sliced)
- **Directions:**

1. Put all the ingredients into a one-quart glass jar and press them with a wooden spoon or muddler, twisting it slightly until the fruit begins to release its juices. Don't pulverize the fruit into pieces.

2. If you plan to drink all or most of the fruit water within the next five hours, fill the jar halfway with ice and then top the jar off with cold drinking water. If you're planning to store the water for longer than five hours before drinking it, fill the jar three-quarters full of ice before topping it off with water.

3. Stir with a chopstick or long spoon and put a lid on the jar. Stick the jar in the fridge to chill, preferably for at least three hours.

4. Strain the water before serving.

Hibiscus Watermelon

Ingredients:

- 2 hibiscus tea bags
- 10 raspberries
- 4 watermelon pieces

Directions:

1. Bring a half quart of water to a boil and then remove it from heat. Put the tea bags into a jar and pour the hot water over them. Steep for ten minutes, then remove the tea bags and let the water cool.

2. Put the fruit into a separate one-quart jar. Press the fruit with a muddle or wooden spoon until the juice starts to release from the fruit. Don't pulverize the fruit.

3. Pour the cooled tea into the jar of fruit and fill the jar with ice, topping it with water. Put a lid on the jar and stick it in the fridge for at least three hours.

4. Strain the water before serving.

Conclusion

Thank you again for downloading this book!

I hope this book was able to help you to in making some of the most delicious and healthful fruit-infused vitamin water recipes on the planet.

The next step is to make infused fruit water a regular part of your life, taking control of your own needs for beverages rather than depending upon commercial products that often contain harmful additives.

Recipe Sources Used in this Book

[1] The Yummy Life .com

[2] Uncommon Designs .com

[3] Everyday Roots .com

[4] Garden Betty .com

[5] The Sweeter the Juice .com

[6] Lose Weight by eating .com

[7] Pharmacology Organics .blogspot.com

[8] Black Doctor .org

[9] Jess Ainscough .com

[10] Bembu .com

[11] She is my Nutritionist .com

[12] Macrobiotic .About.com

[13] Fruit-infused Water: 70 Vitamin Recipes to Finally Cure Tasteless H2O

Preview of "DASH Diet Action Plan Recipes Cookbook: Over 40 Mouthwatering Recipes to Help You Lose Weight, Lower Blood Pressure and Feel Amazing"

The DASH diet plan is rich in vegetables, fruit, nuts, low-fat dairy, fish, poultry, lean meats and whole grains. DASH features high levels of fiber, calcium, magnesium and potassium, as well as low-to-moderate levels of fat. By limiting your sodium and saturated fats, it helps to avoid many health problems like hypertension, obesity and high blood pressure. So the DASH diet is not a temporary crash diet to help you lose weight, but it's a permanent diet you can stay on for your whole life to improve your total health outlook.

The DASH diet is endorsed by:

1. The American Heart Association (AHA)
2. The National Heart, Lung and Blood Institute
3. The Mayo Clinic
4. The 2010 Dietary Guidelines for Americans
5. The 2011 Treatment Guidelines for Women

This book not only offers you a variety of delicious and healthy recipes, but also provides a nutritional analysis of each recipe that—unlike some of its predecessors—includes important factors like the amounts of fat, protein, carbohydrates, sodium, calories and cholesterol. The instructions are easy-to-follow and the recipes are versatile enough for you to make substitutions like exchanging whole wheat flour for all-purpose flour, if you'd like. And this book fits perfectly into your busy schedule, because all the dishes only take about a half-hour or less to make.

Breakfast Recipes

It's Monday morning, you are rushing, and you don't have time to whip a full hearty meal for breakfast? With the DASH Diet Breakfast recipes, you will need just 30-40 minutes to prepare a satisfying, delicious and healthy meal to start the day! Some of the recipes can also be prepared well in advance so you can just pop it in a microwave in the morning, and you're good to go!

Cinnamon French Toast

This delicious recipe can serve as one of your breakfast mainstays, because it has less than a gram of saturated fat, only 2 grams of total fat and only 1 mg of cholesterol. You can substitute any type of bread for the cinnamon bread.

Ready in 35 minutes.

2 Servings

Ingredients

- 4 egg whites
- 1 teaspoon vanilla
- 1/8 teaspoon ground nutmeg
- 4 slices cinnamon bread
- ¼ teaspoon ground cinnamon
- 2 teaspoons powdered sugar

- ¼ cup maple syrup

Directions

1. Whisk the egg whites, vanilla and nutmeg in a small bowl, mixing evenly.

2. Dip each piece of bread into the mix, making sure to coat both sides.

3. Pre-heat a non-stick frying pan or griddle until a drop of water sizzles when you drop it into the pan.

4. Set the bread in the pan and sprinkle cinnamon on it. Cook 4-5 minutes per side, until golden brown.

5. Set the finished bread on a pre-warmed plate and add a teaspoon of powdered sugar and 2 tablespoons of maple syrup to each piece. Serve at once.

Nutritional Analysis (Per Serving)

Calories: 295

Protein: 12 g

Total fat: 2 g

Carbohydrates: 56 g

Sodium: 395 mg

Cholesterol: 1 mg

To download the rest of this book, please click on the following link:

http://www.amazon.com/DASH-Diet-Action-Recipes-Cookbook-ebook/dp/B00KJ79RF8

Check Out My Other Books

If you're interested in finding my other books that are popular on Amazon and Kindle, simply click on the following link:

Below you'll find some of my other books that are popular on Amazon and Kindle as well. Simply click on the links below to check them out.

- "Dash Diet Action Plan and Recipes for Busy People: Lose Weight, Lower Blood Pressure and Feel Amazing!

    - http://www.amazon.com/Dash-Diet-Action-Recipes-People-ebook/dp/B00G07D694

- "DASH Diet Action Plan Recipes Cookbook: Over 40 Mouthwatering Recipes to Help You Lose Weight, Lower Blood Pressure and Feel Amazing"

    - http://www.amazon.com/DASH-Diet-Action-Recipes-Cookbook-ebook/dp/B00KJ79RF8

- "The DASH Diet Action Plan Cookbook for Beginners: A 7-Day Quick Start Guide to Losing Weight, Lowering Blood Pressure and Feeling Amazing: Dash Diet Cookbook, Dash Diet for Weight Loss, Recipes"

    - http://www.amazon.com/DASH-Diet-Action-Cookbook-Beginners-ebook/dp/B00KL1DJ24

If the links do not work, for whatever reason, you can simply search for these titles on the Amazon website to find them.

Offer for Free Books

If you're interested in receiving updates on new books and free book promotions, please click the link below:

https://docs.google.com/forms/d/1ttDqtdRjOeAEtA-BKnq5Hw668vjQSoVWcXCGQ8z9frA/viewform

One Last Thing

Thank you again for downloading this book!

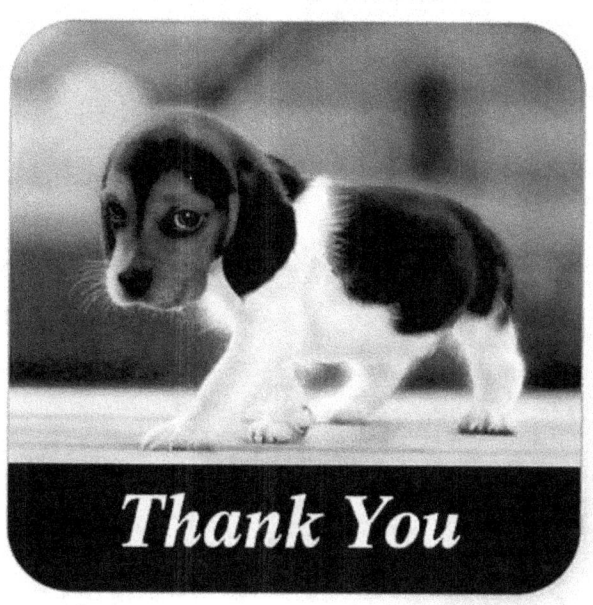

If you enjoyed this book or feel that it has helped you in anyway, then could you please take a minute and post an honest review about it on Amazon?

Your review will help get my book out there to more people and they'll be forever grateful, as will I.

www.ingramcontent.com/pod-product-compliance
Lightning Source LLC
Chambersburg PA
CBHW071420070526
44578CB00003B/635